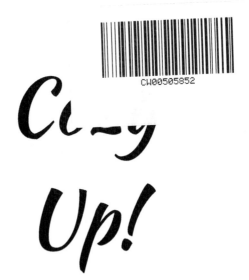

Cosy Up!

How to Thrive During the Coldest Months of the Year

JENNIFER MELVILLE

Table of Contents

Introduction

Hello! Thank you so much for picking up this little book of mine. I'm looking forward to settling in for a cozy chat, and I hope you are too! Although we've likely never met, my guess is we may share a common connection—our love/hate relationship with Old Man Winter! To be fair, winter is a sneaky charmer…a Casanova of sorts! It seduces us with its dazzling beauty one moment, only to knock us off our feet and plow us into a snowbank the next.

Does winter get you down? Do you ever wish you could crawl into a cave and hibernate until spring? I will admit to times I've greeted winter with a heavy heart and defeatist attitude. There's no doubt, winter can be a long, dark, and lonely season. On the bright side, it can also be a time of cozy connection, contemplation, and rest. Over the years, I've learned to shift my perspective and welcome winter with open arms. I'm confident you can too!

As a Canadian who has weathered her fair share of winter storms, I consider myself an unofficial expert on the matter of winter survival. In fact, my goal is to not just survive winter, but to *thrive* and *flourish* during this underrated time of the year. I've come to realize that how you experience winter is more about mindset than the weather forecast!

This book is my recipe for cozy winter living! When seasoned properly, with a sprinkling of positivity and a few extra layers, winter is indeed a delicious time of year. I look forward to sharing my tasty ideas with you on how to make the most of the frosty and frigid days ahead.

This book is meant to be a light, fun and cozy read. View it as a petite source of inspiration to set you up for a successful winter. Savour it in inspiring tidbits, one chapter at a time, or snuggle up on the couch and devour it cover to cover.

Are you ready to *cozy up*!? Grab yourself a steaming cup of your favorite hot drink and let's get started!

1

Tune Into the Magic of Music

Have you ever heard of the phenomenon known as *Blue Monday*? I'm not sure what kind of science was used when coining this term, but the third Monday of January is considered by some to be the most depressing day of the year. Apparently, this is the magical moment when the holiday hangover comes into full effect. Combine a bucket load of Christmas bills, a shovel full of crappy weather, and a hefty serving of low motivation, and you've got a potent recipe for the blues.

Let's imagine for a moment that *today* is *Blue Monday*. You just got home from a frenzied day at work. The winter sun set long before you pull your salt-encrusted vehicle into the garage, weary from a nerve-wracking commute on icy roads.

After changing out of your work clothes and slipping into a sumptuous pair of cashmere leggings and matching sweatshirt, you pull out your phone and hit play on your personalized *Cozy Up!* playlist. As the first few magical notes fill the airwaves, you exhale a blissful sigh. The stress of the day melts away as you find yourself enveloped in the rose-colored sound of your favorite comfort songs. Unlike many people, and against the odds, you are *not* singing the blues on this frosty January evening. You have tapped into the transformative power of music to extinguish negative energy and lift your spirits. Just like a soothing balm, the music comforts your soul, leaving you feeling safe, warm, contented and cozy.

Wait…what's that you say? You don't have a personalized *Cozy Up!* playlist to pull out in case of emergency? Not to worry, I've got you covered. As the saying goes, "Sharing is caring." I'm more than happy to offer my personal suggestion of songs to get you started. I've created a custom *Cozy Up!* playlist and have made it available to everyone on *Spotify*. To access it, just type *Jennifer Melville Author* in *Spotify*'s search box and you should be able to find my account.

Use my selection as a starting point and massage the list to suit your personal taste. Tune into your playlist any time you need to escape the humdrum and darkness that accompanies the season. Conjure up a blissful and cozy mindset while cooking dinner, soaking in the tub, lazing on the couch, and sipping a warm drink at your favorite coffee shop. Immerse yourself in the music and embrace the quiet and contemplative nature of this magical time of the year.

I turn to music regularly to manifest my dreams and alter my mood and mindset. I first sat down to write this book during the height of summer on a hot, humid August afternoon. While my external environment wasn't particularly inspiring, I used music to create a more suitable internal landscape. After reviewing my notes and outlining the chapters, I kicked off the project by creating my *Cozy Up!* playlist. I ran these songs on repeat throughout the entire writing process! My playlist provided the perfect background for inspired writing. (I also wrote a book called *Blissful Christmas* to the sound of *Jingle Bells* in July!)

In case you don't have access to *Spotify*, here is a list of the songs included:

1. *Jardin d'hiver*-Keren Ann
2. *Snowfall*-Ingrid Michaelson
3. *Banana Pancakes*-Jack Johnson
4. *Winter Moon*-Mindy Gledhill
5. *Feels Like Home*-Chantal Kreviazuk
6. *Quiet Nights*-Diana Krall
7. *Cardigan*-Taylor Swift
8. *Wintertime*-Norah Jones
9. *Autumn Town Leaves*-Iron & Wine
10. *Winter Song*-The Head and the Heart
11. *Cold Outside*-Ruth Moody
12. *Cranberry Garden*-Peter Sandberg
13. *Warm Cold Hands*-Peter Sandberg, Jake Isaac
14. *Home*-Edith Whiskers
15. *Under a Smiling Moon*-Peter Sandberg

16. *Song for a Winter's Night*-Sarah McLachlan

17. *January Hymn*-The Decemberists

18. *SnowTime*-James Taylor

Tune in and *cozy up!*

2

Plant a Winter Garden

*I*f you have read any of my other books, you will
know that I am a lifelong Francophile with a
fervent adoration for all things French! (If you
share my passion, I recommend you check out my
title, *Paris in my Panties*.) French food, fashion, art, history,
cinema, music…I love it all! It's therefore no surprise
that the song *Jardin d'hiver* holds the top spot on my
Cozy Up! playlist from the previous chapter. In fact,
this song provided the initial spark of inspiration for
the concept of this book. I played it on repeat last
November for days on end, submersing myself in the
make-believe world of my very own enchanted winter

garden. (And yes, of course, I've got it playing in the background at this very moment!)

If you haven't already listened to this track, I encourage you to tune in. If you don't speak French, google the translated English lyrics so you can follow along and absorb the song's eloquently worded message. My interpretation of this song is that it represents the author's vision of a sacred space where she can retreat during the winter (or tough times) to soothe both her body and soul. It is a place of comfort, beauty, and solace where she is surrounded by all her favorite things. Its inviting atmosphere serves to shelter her from the external world and all its unpleasantries. Her winter garden includes everything from glowing lights and teapots to lace and seaside photographs. It certainly sounds like a dreamy little hideaway!

I think each and every one of us needs and deserves a winter garden of our own. The great news is that you don't need access to soil or water to grow this kind of garden, you can plant it wherever you like. All your winter garden needs to grow and thrive is a little TLC on your part.

Think of a space in your home where you enjoy spending time, one that serves as a refuge from the stressors and obligations of the outside world. This might be a little reading nook where you can pass away the hours lost in a captivating book. It might be your bathroom, where you enjoy long soaks in the tub, immersing yourself in fragrant bubbles. It might be your kitchen, where you love to experiment with new recipes. It might be your closet, where you love to play dress-up with all your lovely clothes and accessories. Now ask yourself, what little touches of beauty and comfort can you add to your garden space to make it more inviting? What would you like to surround yourself with to shield yourself from the harsh reality of winter? It might be a table lamp for softer lighting, a fuzzy throw to warm up your legs, a cheerful potted plant, a deliciously scented candle, or even a wireless speaker so you can play background music. (Of course, I recommend the *Cozy Up!* playlist.) You might want to decorate it with a basket of seashells to remind you of the sunny beach days to come. Have fun coming up with little touches to upgrade your space and

transform it into your personalized winter getaway…
no plane ticket required.

My *jardin d'hiver* is my bedroom. It is such a soothing
and relaxing space to retreat to any time of the day.
Last year my husband and I invested in a new mattress,
and it is divine! I've dressed it in a high-quality set of
cotton percale sheets that feel like butter on my skin.
I love crawling into bed early on cold winter nights,
snuggling under the covers while I read or write in my
journal. We recently removed my husband's home
office desk from the corner (leftover from the Covid
era) and replaced it with a comfortable leather reading
chair. I've decorated the room with seashells, candles,
and sentimental artwork. Our bedroom feels like a
secret getaway that we have all to ourselves…no kids
allowed! (Dogs, on the other hand, are more than
welcome. I outfitted the space with a couple of fluffy
dog beds so my little poodles Coco and Junior can
join me in the garden.)

Keep in mind, a winter garden doesn't have to be
a physical space. It can come in the form of a mindset
and a way of living. You can carry a winter garden in

your heart, so that it is always available to uplift your spirits. For instance, in *Jardin d'hiver*, the songstress chooses to wear the unexpected choice of a feminine floral dress on a rainy November day. You can do the same, by reaching for things that bring you joy and uplift your spirits. It might be spritzing yourself in your favorite perfume, reaching for the silk and lace lingerie to wear under your jeans, or treating yourself to a decadent hot chocolate instead of your regular morning coffee.

It's all up to you to plant the seeds in your winter garden. Happy sowing!

3

Revamp Your Skincare Routine

*A*re you feeling a bit parched after a glorious but sizzling summer? If there is one part of our bodies that breathes a sigh of relief when the summer sun dims, it is our *skin*. Despite my best efforts with sunscreen during the hottest months, I know the sun's sneaky rays still sink their way into the layers of my skin, doing a number on my DNA!

I'm in my late forties and spent a great deal of my youth worshipping the sun, (as much as that's even possible living in Canada). Maybe you can relate? Even though the summers of my past were short, I jumped at any opportunity to work on my tan. Decades later, I'm paying the price for my bad habits with a peppering of dark spots on my face.

The arrival of cooler temperatures offers a welcome opportunity to regroup and refocus in the skincare department. It actually feels like a relief to say farewell to the intensity of the summer sun and allow our skin to take a breather. It's time to reconnect with our skin, allowing us to kick off the new season with a radiant complexion.

Pull out the mirror and take a good look at your skin after a thorough cleansing. Do you have problem areas that could use a little extra TLC? Is your skin feeling dehydrated? Are your pores plugged after months of slathering on heavy sunscreen? Has a new crop of dark spots surfaced across your forehead? Identify your concerns and then come up with a game plan to address them.

A dip in temperature marks a good time to schedule a facial (do-it-yourself or at the spa). I always like to check in with my esthetician when the seasons change.

I look to her for advice on what products would best suit my skincare needs. This past fall I underwent a gentle clinical face peel. The results were amazing. It removed an unsightly layer of summer sludge from my skin and left me with a glowing complexion.

Sort through your skincare products, swapping summer friendly items for those best suited for cooler temperatures. Depending on the dryness of your skin, this usually means moving to a heavier moisturizer, or switching your gel cleanser with a creamier version. I always look forward to pulling out my retinol cream as the sun cools off. Retinol is a powerful beauty tool that tackles several skincare concerns including hyper-pigmentation, acne, fine lines and wrinkles. That being said, it isn't for everyone. Those with sensitive skin may need to avoid it. If your skin can handle it, experts usually recommend you avoid sun exposure when using retinol, so the timing is perfect.

Give yourself the gift of a glowing complexion and head into the cooler months feeling fresh-faced and confident.

4

Be a Kid Again

T here is a lot of whining, lamenting, grumbling, and rumbling that goes on when the mercury drops. I'll be the first to admit that I do my fair share of complaining about the woes of winter. (My husband can attest to this!) Visions of hefty heating bills, salt-stained boots, and windshields varnished in thick layers of ice leave many adults feeling defeated and exhausted before the first snowflake even hits the ground. Kids, on the other hand, seem to approach all seasons with an enviable carefree attitude. What if we ditched our gloomy adult lenses and opted to view winter through the eyes of a child?

Children approach winter with a sense of wonder and enthusiasm. Instead of lamenting slushy sidewalks, they luxuriate in the deliciousness of snow days. They snuggle deeper under the covers as they savour the sweetness of an unexpected day off. They marvel at the dazzling beauty of a fresh snowfall as they scramble to bundle up their bodies and tug on heavy snow boots. They venture outdoors, oblivious to time and temperature, rolling snowballs and giggling with friends. They fly down ski slopes with rosy cheeks, squealing with laughter when they fumble and fall. They seek solitude under the snow-laden branches of an evergreen, slowly sipping hot chocolate out of a thermos. Instead of resisting the season, they immerse themselves in it and all the magic it has to offer.

Let's take a moment to indulge in a little reminiscing. Close your eyes and think back to some of your fondest childhood winter memories. What did you do for fun? What did you enjoy most about the chilliest months of the year? Did you participate in winter sports and activities like skating, skiing, and sledding? Did you ever go ice fishing with your dad? Did you build snow forts with the neighborhood kids? Did you spend your free time cozied up at the dining room table doing crafts with your sister? Did you spend Saturday afternoons helping your mom in the kitchen, chopping vegetables for her famous chili?

Once you've had time to reflect, pick one or two of your winter favorites, and commit to indulging in them this season…no excuses. Make it your intention to have some real *fun* this winter, whatever that looks like for you.

I spent countless hours outdoors during my childhood winters. I lived down the street from an outdoor skating rink, and had the woods as my backyard, where I snowshoed with my family. My idea of winter fun is getting out and enjoying nature, no matter the weather. I make a point of walking the forest trails around my home every single day. It helps that I have my little dog Coco to motivate me. He loves to run, and as you'd expect from a style-conscious poodle, he owns a fashionable collection of winter wear to keep him snug. I also picked up skiing again in adulthood, which is something I really enjoyed growing up.

Having winter specific activities to look forward to helps add a spark of child-like excitement to the season. What's on your agenda?

5

Ease Into Mornings

As the days grow shorter, mornings get rougher. Long gone are those energizing 6 a.m. sunrises. You'll be lucky if you see the sun peek over the horizon before you leave for work!

Be gentle with yourself. Your body is confused, wondering why it's being roused from slumber while the stars still light the night sky. It's not easy to drag yourself out from under the covers when shrouded in a cloak of darkness. The struggle is real!

I consider myself a morning person and have always been an early riser. That being said, even I need a little coaxing to greet the day with a smile this time of year. Having a gentle morning routine that eases me into the day with kindness definitely helps.

Do you naturally wake up to the rhythm of your internal clock, or are you usually jolted from dreamland by a screeching alarm? I despise alarm clocks! Even the high-tech ringtones on my smartphone send my body into fight or flight mode. It's no fun waking up in a panic. My husband and I came up with a much kinder solution. We invested in a fancy alarm clock that simulates the rising of the sun, complete with the sound of birds chirping in the background. In my view, it offers a more civilized way to wake up! You can find these light alarm clocks on *Amazon* for a reasonable price. (I will warn you, teenagers may be immune to their effects. It scored a failing mark on waking up my sixteen-year-old!)

I sometimes tune into a guided morning meditation while I'm still snuggled under the covers. It's a calming way to rouse myself from sleep. My favorite is called *Morning Meditation for Mothers* by Fleur Chambers, which is available for free on the *Insight Timer* app. If you are someone who likes lingering in bed for a few extra minutes, you may find this type of meditation enjoyable.

Indulging in a warm and soothing breakfast is another way to kick off a winter's morn on the right foot. As soon as the weather cools, I swap my summer breakfast of yogurt, granola, and berries for a hearty bowl of oatmeal topped with poached pears and cinnamon. I usually precook a pot for the week and reheat my servings to help save time. Have fun playing around with tasty toppings to keep things interesting. Nuts, seeds, spices, dried fruit, and even dark chocolate can be sprinkled on top for added flavour and nutrition.

Most of us rely on either tea or coffee for a morning pick-me-up. Why not play barista and experiment with concocting an exciting new morning beverage? While visiting Paris last fall, I had the most delicious matcha hot chocolate at a little café called *Saint Pearl*. (If you are lucky enough to visit the City of Light, it is located on la rue des Saints-Pères in the heart of Saint-Germain-des Prés.) When I came home, I made it my mission to replicate the recipe. I indulged in this treat often last winter, savouring the taste of Paris on the coldest of Canadian mornings.

Give yourself a cozy hug of kindness this winter and ease into your days feeling loved and uplifted.

6

Be Jeweled

I treated myself to a pedicure today, even though sandal season has long since passed. Although my toes are mostly under wraps this time of year, they still appreciate donning a pretty coat. I opted for a deep ruby red, which adds a bit of sparkle to my step.

Treat yourself to a little color therapy this fall and winter by incorporating jewel tones into your personal style. Jewel tones are rich, vibrant, and luxurious. Diamonds aren't our only friends. I consider rubies, emeralds, sapphires, and garnets as members of my inner circle as well! These highly saturated colors add some much-needed vibrancy to dull, grey winter days.

As the curtain falls on summer, a wardrobe change is in order. It's time to pack away the airy sundresses in favor of fabulous denim, snuggly sweaters, and elegantly tailored wool coats. It's also the perfect opportunity to shake up your color palette by embracing deeper, richer, and darker hues. I know many of us like to play it safe by filling our closets with black, black and more black, (in my case it's navy, navy and more navy) but there's always room for a little color here and there. If you aren't ready to commit to a bright emerald green sweater, start small. Incorporate the jewel tones into your accessories. When I was in Paris last fall, I purchased a sumptuous cashmere scarf in a shade of deep cranberry red. It pairs perfectly with my classic navy coat, and gives my complexion a rosy, wintry glow (and hopefully a hint of French girl style).

You can also add more drama and mystery to your seasonal look by playing around with your makeup routine. I'm a minimalist when it comes to most areas of life, and makeup is no exception. While I tend to stick to natural-looking cosmetics, I do like the look of a sultry red lip during the cooler months. I've had a tube of *Clinique's Almost Lipstick* in *Black Honey* in my cosmetic bag for more years than I can count. This cult classic was launched in 1971 and is one of those products that is flattering on everyone. As Janet Pardo, Senior Vice President of Product Development at *Clinique* says, "It's magical. It makes your teeth look whiter, it makes your lips look gorgeous, and it's very forgiving—you don't even need a mirror when you put it on. It's functional, yet so desirable."

There are so many stunning jewel-toned nail polishes on the market, I always have a hard time choosing when faced with the generous rack of bottles at the nail salon. Some of them have such great names! If you are a lover of red as I am, you can't go wrong with *OPI's Relentless Ruby*, *Give a Garnet*, or *Bring out the Big Gems*. If you are a bit more adventurous, try out *Blue My Mind*, described as a "sizzling sapphire". Sounds tempting, doesn't it?

What dazzling jewels will you dig out of the treasure chest this winter?

7

Shovel Yourself Out

I kicked off the most recent fall season feeling disheveled and unorganized. After a carefree summer with my teenage boys at home most days, the house was in rough shape. One of my sons made it his summer mission to bulk up on muscle, and as you'd expect, our kitchen became command central. When he wasn't at the gym, or his part-time job at the golf course, he was parked in the kitchen, cooking and eating on repeat.

I felt like I was living with a messy college room-mate that I never signed up for. Don't get me wrong,

I love this boy with all my heart. He is the sweetest of sweethearts with a heart of gold. He's just not the best housekeeper.

My other roomie, his older brother, spent his summer days building a remote-controlled speedboat. Instead of working on this project in his designated basement workshop (he has claimed the entire basement for himself), he chose to set up shop in various locations of our home including our front doorstep, the dining room table, the kitchen counter and even the bathroom.

To be fair to both of them, I made it my summer mission to chill out and cool off on the nagging. I didn't exactly hold them accountable for their messes, and as a result, the house was in a fine state of disarray by the time September rolled around.

I realized that my chaotic internal emotions were really just a reflection of my cluttered and scruffy external environment. The summer season is hard on one's home. With the doors and windows open all the time, so much dirt and debris gets tracked inside. I know a lot of people tend to associate a deep household clean-up with the spring, but I'm a proponent of entering winter on the housekeeping offensive.

The shorter days and chilly temperatures of the season encourage us to bunker down and spend more time indoors. Your home is really your winter retreat. Don't you want this space to feel welcoming, clean, uncluttered, and organized?

I started my fall cleanup at ground zero—the kitchen. Each day I chose one cupboard or drawer to wipe down and declutter. I didn't want the task to feel overwhelming, so I picked away at the mess gently but methodically. The more space I created, the more my mood lifted. My momentum picked up and I eventually paid a visit to every room in our home. I had the most fun in my closet, where I swapped all my summer clothes out with my favorite fall and winter wardrobe pieces. Before storing my warm-weather attire, I made a point of assessing each piece honestly. I ended up selling a bunch of stuff on *Poshmark* and made enough funds to finance a few fall wardrobe additions. There's nothing better than getting paid for your housecleaning efforts!

Get inspired to spruce up your home for the hibernation season that awaits you. Tackling the job in bite-sized pieces makes the task feel achievable instead of overwhelming. Kick off your efforts in your hottest clutter zones; those that irritate you the most.

As you shovel out the physical clutter, the mental clutter will clear as well. You will head into winter feeling organized and super chill (just figuratively of course!)

8

Redefine Comfort Food

*D*inners in the dark have my body craving cozy foods that will warm me up from the inside out. With the days of light summery salads behind us, it is time to shift our menus to meals that satisfy our yearning for warmth and comfort.

Cool temperatures call for some good old-fashioned comfort food, to be sure! That being said, traditional comfort fare is often not the healthiest. I grew up in the seventies and eighties, so I tend to identify comfort food as conventional, North American meat-and-potato-style meals. Shepherd's pie, meatloaf, homemade macaroni and cheese, gooey lasagna, and dishes laden with heavy gravies and sauces are all foods that come to mind.

For many, the heavy nature of cold weather menus often leads to unwanted winter weight gain. An increase in calorie intake coupled with a decrease in activity is rarely a winning combination. The good news is that it is possible to dine in a fashion that is both *comforting* and *healthy*. Grandma's recipes may just need a little tweaking!

Healthy vegetable-laden soups are superstars in my recipe book. Not only do they take off the chill, but they are easy to make, filling to the belly, packed with nutrients and easy on the waistline. A steaming bowl of nourishing soup served with a slice of hearty multigrain bread makes a satisfying meal.

Soup freezes and stores well, which classifies it as a convenience food in my opinion. A large pot of soup can go a long way! Double up on your recipe and build your winter stores by tucking half in the freezer. Instead of opting for a takeout lunch at work, pack yourself a homemade cup of soup that can be quickly reheated in the office microwave.

Have fun experimenting with new recipes and building up a repertoire of healthy soups that you and your family will look forward to on a cold winter's night. To get you started, here is a simple recipe I throw together regularly. It also happens to be my son's favorite. (I aim to please!)

Jen's *Cozy Up!* Soup

- ✓ 2 Tbsp olive oil
- ✓ 1 onion, finely chopped
- ✓ 2 large carrots, peeled and chopped
- ✓ ½ cup of chopped celery
- ✓ 3 medium potatoes, peeled and cubed
- ✓ 8 cups of vegetable broth
- ✓ 1 can of diced tomatoes
- ✓ ½ cup of brown rice
- ✓ ½ cup of brown lentils
- ✓ ½ cup frozen peas
- ✓ 2 tsp thyme
- ✓ salt and pepper to taste

1. Heat the olive oil in a stock pot and add the diced onion, followed by the carrots and celery. Sauté these vegetables until they are tender.
2. Add the vegetable broth, canned tomatoes, potatoes, brown rice and lentils to the pot. Allow the pot to simmer until the potatoes, rice and lentils are cooked.
3. Add the frozen peas, along with the thyme and salt and pepper to taste.
4. Serve and enjoy!

Bon appétit!

9

Be Prepared

Today I'm writing by candlelight, which certainly adds to the cozy atmosphere of my surroundings. On this storm day, with the house quiet and the power out, I have been gifted the perfect backdrop for creativity and inspired writing.

Of course, it's not always easy to look at the positive side of things during inclement weather. I will admit to releasing a loud groan, (ok, a loud wail) when the lights first flickered, then extinguished to darkness. The lack of electricity is an inconvenience in our modern world, as we have all come to rely on it so extensively. Since our house is on a well, no power means no water pumping through our pipes. Although the lack of electricity and water is stressful, my anxious feelings have been dampened by the fact that we took a few measures ahead of the storm to prepare for the worst.

If you were a Girl Guide as I was growing up, you may remember the guiding motto, "Be prepared." Although I didn't realize it at the age of eleven, this was an important life lesson I'm glad was drilled into my head! Being prepared for the challenges that go hand in hand with winter allows us to glide through the season with greater peace of mind. We are able to weather the storms with less anxiety, which in turn allows us to relish the tranquil pause in life that foul weather offers.

Do you have a winter preparedness checklist, or do you usually prefer to wing it and tackle problems as they arise? There are a few simple things you can do to get ahead of the game, and I guarantee, when the snow hits the fan, you'll be happy you put in a little upfront effort.

Have you booked an appointment to put your snow tires on? The first snowfall of the season typically results in numerous vehicle collisions, as unprepared motorists slip and slide in their summer tires. Plan ahead and get your car outfitted for winter well in advance. Service stations book up quickly during the pre-winter season, so it is best to call early.

Stock your vehicle with an extra bottle or two of cold-weather windshield washer fluid, as well as a few extra pairs of mittens and warm hats. Stashing a couple of blankets or an old winter coat in the trunk is also a good idea. I once caught my husband driving around in the dead of winter with my two toddlers strapped into their car seats in nothing but diapers. I hate to imagine what might have happened had they slipped on a patch of ice and gone off the road. (You can guess he didn't think to bring any spare diapers either!)

Keeping your house stocked with the essentials also keeps stress levels low. There are lots of great websites that provide guidance on creating an emergency preparedness kit for your home. Sit down with your family and come up with a plan that suits your needs and circumstances. In the last couple of months, my community in Nova Scotia has experienced several terrifying emergencies ranging from forest fires to flash floods, to hurricanes and nor'easters. With the effects of global warming, extreme weather events are on the rise across the globe. It's something we all need to think about.

So today, while the wind batters my windows, I can sit back and enjoy the solitude. I made sure my laptop battery was juiced up so I could tap out a few chapters of this book. All our phones were fully charged, and our vehicles were topped up with fuel. We have gas on hand for our small generator, and we stocked a half dozen sheets of plywood in case some damage control was in order. Thankfully, it looks like we will make it out of this storm unscathed, but it's always better to be safe than sorry.

Tap into your inner Girl Guide and prepare yourself to greet Old Man Winter with a smile when he comes knocking!

10

Update Your Do

*A*re you a fan of the *Netflix* hit *Emily in Paris*? If you binge-watched your way through all three seasons as I did, you probably remember the scene from season three where Emily chops herself a fresh set of bangs over the bathroom sink. Emily was going through a tumultuous time and her impulsive new bangs, (jokingly referred to as trauma bangs by her friend Mindy) were intended to snap her out of her funk.

Although it is both superficial and simplistic to think a new haircut can solve all your problems, I think

Emily was on to something. There are times in life when a physical change can ignite a spark in your inner landscape. There is nothing quite like a new bold haircut or a dazzling new color job to help reframe both your face and your state of mind.

I experienced the energizing power of a new do last winter when I too decided to take the plunge and outfit myself with a set of February blues bangs. February is always a tough month for me. The crispness of a fresh new year has worn off, the temperatures are frigid, and there are many more weeks of wintry weather booked on the agenda. I had just finished binging on another *Netflix* show, *Wednesday*, and like many fans, fell in love with Jenna Ortega and her character. Yes, Wednesday is dark and a little twisted, but she has a lot of spectacularly positive qualities I admire including confidence, fearlessness, and an amazing sense of deadpan humour. I found myself wondering if a new set of bangs à la Wednesday Addams would allow some of her self-assuredness to rub off on me!

I toyed with the idea for a couple of weeks, admittedly scared to take the leap. After all, the last time I sported bangs was 1988. *Traumatic bangs* would accurately describe them (think 80's teased). I finally decided to surrender to the scissors when my sixteen-year-old spoke the honest truth— "Just get the bangs Mom. Like, you've had the same haircut your entire life!" Ouch!

So off I trotted to the hair salon, my Jenna Ortega *Pinterest* board in hand. Twenty minutes later I walked out of the salon feeling like a brand new woman, wondering what took me so long to shake things up. My new look left me feeling inspired and empowered. It was just the boost I needed to brave the rest of the winter. I dove into a few new creative projects and crossed off several items that were gathering dust on my to-do list. The fact that my son told me I looked ten years younger was the cherry on top!

If you've got a case of the winter blues, a sassy new hairdo might just provide the jolt of excitement you need to improve your mood and your outlook. Practically speaking, after a summer full of sunshine, salt and chlorine, your hair could probably benefit from a solid trim and a deep condition. Why not take the opportunity to give yourself a fresh new look?

Have a peek in the mirror. How long have you had your current hairstyle? Do my son's harsh words ring true for you too? Have you been considering bangs yourself, or maybe a new dramatic color? What if you chopped your shoulder-length style into an edgy chin-length bob? Maybe you don't have a particular style in mind but crave change. Tap into some of that Wednesday bravery and give your stylist a carte blanche. It's only hair, so nothing is permanent!

Give your hair and your attitude a makeover this winter with a bold new do!

11

Light Your Fire

*A*re you familiar with the term *glamping*? If not, you can probably guess its meaning. It represents a combination of the words *glamorous* and *camping*. I was surprised to see this trendy phenomenon included in the Oxford Dictionary, which describes glamping as, "A form of camping that involves accommodation and facilities more luxurious than those associated with traditional camping." I'm not exaggerating when I say that many winter mornings at my house have glamping vibes. You know that feeling when your bladder is bursting, but you can't bring yourself to crawl out of your sleeping bag to pee in the freezing cold? That would be me on many a winter morning when the thermostat reads 14°C (57°F). The only difference is that I am apparently living in a modern home, and not a flimsy tent! (We load our woodstove every night, but by morning it's due for a refill.)

The current economic climate has forced most households to rein in their energy consumption. Heat costs money! As an accountant, I appreciate a good cost-saving strategy. That being said, my husband and I hold differing opinions on what constitutes a comfortable room temperature. Mr. Metabolism, as I've nicknamed him, runs on high octane, and I apparently run on regular unleaded.

Let's be honest, it's no fun feeling cold. I personally turn to stone (or ice rather) when I am physically cold, which means my productivity around the house comes to a grinding halt. It's hard to feel your best or get anything accomplished when you are curled in the fetal position, hiding under a heap of blankets!

Ignite a fire from within and boost your metabolism by working up a sweat. Nothing warms me up better than physical activity. People in general tend to be less active during the cooler months as they spend more time indoors. This doesn't have to be the case, as winter offers a great opportunity to move your workouts inside. During the coldest of months, I rely on my morning workout to thaw both my body and brain.

I'm a huge fan of at-home workouts because they are convenient, flexible, and readily available to everyone. There are so many options out there, from paid streaming services to freebies on *YouTube*. I've been a fan of *BODi* (formerly *Beachbody*) for almost a decade, so I can unequivocally recommend their programs. They offer something for everyone including yoga, Pilates, dance, cardio, weightlifting and more. I'm currently working my way through a series called *Sure Thing* with Megan Davies. She is positive and upbeat, and I'm always toasty and energized after spending thirty minutes with her.

Stoke your inner fire and get moving this winter. Just like a hot bed of coals, you will be glowing!

12

Exercise Your Green Thumb

A number of years ago, our family held a CSA subscription with a local farm. CSA is short for Community Supported Agriculture. It is a model that connects farmers and consumers directly. Each week we received a share of produce from the farm. During times of bounty, the box was overflowing with fresh veggie goodness. During leaner times on the farm (the winter!), the box was a little less inspiring. While I do try to eat in season as much as possible, by the time late February rolled around, I'd had my fill of turnip. I knew I was getting desperate the day I presented a turnip cake to my family and tried to pass it off as dessert.

Give your winter diet a boost of color by exercising your green thumb. Indoor gardening is an easy and rewarding way to infuse your body with a wide array of vitamins and minerals. What can you grow in your living room or on your kitchen counter you may ask? Sprouts of course!

Spouts are one of the easiest foods to grow, (spoken by someone who has failed miserably in many gardening endeavors). They require very little equipment and very little space. I grow mine in a simple jar-style sprouter, but there are more elaborate setups you can purchase, depending on the volume you want to produce. In less than a week, your sprouts will be ready to harvest and enjoy! They make great additions to sandwiches and salads, satisfying our body's craving for freshness.

Growing microgreens is another fun option. While sprouts are germinated seeds, microgreens are basically baby plants. Microgreens are grown in trays of soil, so require more space and equipment. They take a little longer to grow than sprouts (usually around three weeks), but their tender leaves are worth the wait. It's nice to stagger your planting to help ensure a continuous supply.

If you are interested in partaking in some winter gardening, there are many online resources available to get you started. One of my favorite sources for seeds, supplies and information is a company called *Mumm's Sprouting Seeds*, which can be found at www.sprouting.com. They carry a huge selection of organic seeds and ship to both the United States and Canada.

Of course, you don't need to stick with the edible variety of indoor gardening. You can also fill your plate with food for the soul—indoor houseplants. Apparently, the popularity of houseplants skyrocketed during the pandemic, and it seems there is no sign of a slowdown. As I write today, the hashtag #plantsmakepeoplehappy has 12,238,531 posts on *Instagram*! If you haven't jumped on this bandwagon already, winter is the perfect time to invite more greenery into your home. Plants provide a breath of fresh air from the bleak winter landscape. There is also something soothing and therapeutic about tending to plants and caring for another living thing.

I'm partial to succulent varieties. They are low maintenance, drought resistant and come in so many interesting shapes and colors. I also enjoyed overwintering my potted geraniums indoors last year. Geraniums are considered annuals in my hardiness zone. Their brilliant red blooms are a fleeting summer treat. I have a photo of these beauties in full bloom last March, with a snowstorm raging in the background!

13

Hit the Trail

As members of the animal kingdom, it is instinctively tempting to nestle into our caves for the winter and hibernate the days away. Although this sounds enticing, too much time spent indoors can lead to a crummy case of cabin fever. Staying connected with the natural world is simultaneously calming and energizing, no matter the season.

During the sizzling summer months, the ocean beckons us to its salty shores. We humans flock to the sea in droves to cool our bodies and soothe our souls. We savour the briny air and sigh with relief as the refreshing waters wash away our worries. When the temperatures plunge, it is the forest that summons us. With harsh weather on the horizon, it knows that it can provide a safe place of retreat when the winter winds howl.

There is no denying, it can be tough to find the motivation to peel yourself away from the cozy warmth of your cabin and plunge yourself into the hostile winter environment. Despite the unpleasantries of winter, (sleet, snow, biting winds and subzero temperatures) I still try to venture outside at least once a day. What I've discovered over the years is that no matter how nasty the weather, the forest is my happy place.

When my face is being whipped by a -20 windchill, I seek refuge amongst the trees. Their sturdy branches lovingly shield me from the harsh wind. When my tank is on empty and I've grown weary of the darkness, I duck onto a wooded trail. The forest offers a warm welcome and dazzles me with its enchanting beauty. When my mind is racing, I seek solitude under a canopy of snow-laden spruce. The trees buffer the commotion and offer quiet comfort and escape.

Get outside! Seek comfort and joy in the company of trees. Include a wintry hike on your weekend agenda. Escape the office for an invigorating zip through the nearby park on your lunch break. Energize yourself with an early morning wander through the backyard.

Wintertime is the optimal season for taking advantage of your local hiking trails and wooded city parks. There is a positive side to the weather this time of year. You can marvel at the beauty of the winter landscape without the nuisance of bugs, crowds, and oppressive heat. As long as you bundle up, the conditions are ideal. On particularly cold days I slip a set of hand warmers in my mittens and a thermos of hot cocoa in my knapsack. These extra measures allow me to enjoy the scenery a little longer and soak up an extra dose of vitamin D.

Can you hear the forest? It's calling your name!

14

Dress for the Weather

The other day my toy poodle Junior and I were walking in a local park when we crossed paths with a sizeable Samoyed. The sight of this striking animal stopped us both in our tracks, but for very different reasons. Weighing in at less than five pounds, Junior has developed a spicy case of *little dog syndrome* over the years. He defiantly puffed out his chest, blocked the Samoyed's path and dared the towering giant to make the next move. I, on the other hand, was starstruck as I swooned over this exquisite creature's luxurious coat. While Junior scurried away in a snit, I mentally added a snow-white coat to my winter wardrobe wish list!

When it comes to braving the elements, one key component of your wardrobe deserves special attention and consideration—outerwear. Thankfully, as our fluffy white friend (or foe in Junior's opinion) so brilliantly demonstrated, you don't need to sacrifice style to stay toasty and warm. There is plenty of room for both function and fashion in your winter wardrobe.

That Samoyed trotted on the trail proudly with his head held high. He looked amazing, and he *knew* it! Fortunately, you too can sport a coat that makes you look and feel fabulous. Choose something polished and pulled together instead of frumpy and dumpy. If you want to elevate your style this winter, nothing beats a *tailored coat*. More likely than not, you already have a stunner hiding in the back of your closet. That elegant wool dress coat need not be saved for special occasions. Drape it over a pair of jeans and a woolly sweater for a casually chic winter look.

If you don't own a tailored coat, add one to your wish list and start saving your pennies. Coats tend to be expensive. They are investment pieces that should be chosen carefully so you can enjoy them for many winters to come. With so many styles available, (belted, single-breasted, double-breasted, cocoon, fit and flare…etc.) you won't have trouble finding an option that flatters your unique shape. I recommend sticking with classic cuts and colors that won't fall out of style. I own a timeless navy peacoat with shiny gold buttons that I've had for over six years. I still get excited each year when the temperatures drop and I get to pull it out of storage. It has the power to turn any outfit from drab to fab!

Be sure to top off your sophisticated new coat with a few fun accessories. Not only do hats, scarves, gloves, and mittens keep us warm, but they also come in a zillion different colors, patterns, and styles. This is where the real winter fun begins. While I usually stick with neutrals like black, navy, grey and camel, I'm willing to take more risks when it comes to accessorizing. There's nothing like a pop of red to add some fiery spice to a winter outfit. Choose *your* favorite color and wrap yourself in its uplifting coziness.

Lastly, if you are going to strut your stuff this winter, you need to put your best foot (or boot) forward. When it comes to winter footwear, it goes beyond style and warmth. Safety is paramount. Icy conditions turn sidewalks and parking lots into treacherous landscapes! I've been that foolish girl slithering my way through winter in a fabulous but impractical pair of leather-soled boots. (By the way, one looks less than fabulous sitting on one's butt in the middle of the mall parking lot.) Rugged conditions call for rugged soles. Tuck your cute fall booties away in favor of a solid pair of boots that will help you maintain your vertical position this winter! I've since upgraded to a proper pair of boots with thick, rubbery treads. I was able to snag a preloved pair on *Poshmark* from the Montreal-based company *Pajar*. Although their products are pricey, you can trust a Canadian company to do winter boots right. They even offer an entire line of boots with built-in ice grippers!

Envelope yourself in elegance this winter and elevate both your attitude and your style!

15

Tuck Yourself In

'*T*is the season when many animals are nestled all snug in their burrows, passing the
long months of winter in a deep state of hibernation. While we as humans don't officially hibernate, we do tend to slow down in the winter. As the
days grow shorter and daylight wanes, it is natural for
our bodies to crave more sleep.

Tune into the messages your body is sending. If
it is asking for more rest, it's quite possible it *needs* more
downtime. Evenings are a time to soften and recharge
our energy stores for the following day. Set yourself

up for a long winter's nap by adopting an evening routine that focuses on relaxation and self-care.

When the supper dishes are done in my house, that usually means one thing…it's *jammy time*! Even though bedtime isn't for a few hours, I like to lounge in comfort during my downtime. Winter calls for cozy pajamas and fluffy slippers! Cozy, of course, doesn't have to mean frumpy. Instead of slipping on a pair of old sweats and a ratty t-shirt, outfit yourself with loungewear that makes you look and feel good. I love menswear-style PJ sets for the winter. The matching long-sleeved shirts and pants keep you warm, while still allowing you to look stylish and pulled together.

On particularly chilly evenings, look for ways to add some heat to your bedtime routine. When my youngest was little, he used to sleep with a heated stuffed animal. I purchased the doll in an attempt the put an end to the fact I was still sleeping with my eight-year-old. Although the doll never solved this problem (a puppy finally did), it did keep his bed nice and warm. I recently started slipping a microwaveable heating pad under my own covers a few minutes before bedtime. It feels delicious to crawl between warm sheets on a cold night.

Being immersed from head to toe in hot water is a surefire way to take off the chill. Spend your evenings luxuriating in the bathtub. Create an atmosphere that encourages you to exhale your stress by dimming the lights, lighting a candle, and playing soft music. (Yes, I'm plugging my *Cozy Up!* playlist again.)

Warm yourself from the inside out with a soothing cup of bedtime tea. Be sure to avoid caffeinated varieties if you are prone to sleep difficulties. My go-to nighttime brew is a cup of chamomile with a spoonful of honey.

Tuck yourself in with a bedtime story! Travel back to your childhood and cozy up with a bedtime meditation/sleep story. I adore *The Snow Day: Winter Sleep Story by Michelle's Sanctuary* on the *Insight Timer* app. This nostalgic wintry tale, specifically created for adults, sets the scene for a sound and cozy sleep.

Escape to the winter of your dreams by creating a blissful bedtime routine that focuses on warmth, wellness, and relaxation.

16

Awaken Your Senses with Scent

The clean crisp smell of freshly fallen snow, the hint of woodsmoke floating in the air, the tantalizing aroma of sugar cookies fresh from the oven—these are just a few scents that define the cooler months of the year. Our sense of smell is a powerful component of our winter survival toolkit. Of all our senses, it is the one most connected with memories and emotions. You can use this science to your advantage by surrounding yourself with elevating aromas that evoke warm and cozy thoughts and feelings.

Inspired by my plan to write this chapter, I experimented with an interesting mindfulness exercise this morning. During my morning walk in the woods, I focused all my awareness on my sense of smell. As I meandered along the trail, I concentrated on my breathing and the different smells I encountered along the way. This was the first time I really noticed that different areas of the path emitted different scents. (My dog Coco obviously figured this one out long ago!) I took note of the sweet musky smell of rotting leaves, the damp earthy scent of the forest floor, and the fresh green aroma of spruce needles. As I immersed myself in the experience, I was overcome with a feeling of safety. These smells remind me of my father—my protector as a child. He and I spent countless hours together in the woods growing up, so it's no wonder I associate the scents of the forest with the security of his presence.

What pleasant emotions will keep you warm this winter? What fond memories would you like to revisit? Take a moment to reminisce and make a list of some of your favorite winter experiences from the past, along with their associated scents. Did you enjoy baking with your grandmother? Maybe you need to sprinkle a little cinnamon and a splash of vanilla into your life. Do you long to be transported back to your college days, where you philosophized for hours with your friends at the campus coffee shop? The delicious scents of freshly brewed espresso and dark chocolate should do the trick.

Fill your home with your favorite winter memories! I prefer burning candles during the darkest and coldest months, but an essential oil diffuser is another great option. I also love switching my liquid hand soap out with the seasons. I've currently got peppermint vanilla swirl on tap.

As I write today, I'm burning the *Ember & Oak* candle, locally made by a company called *Noël & Co.,* (which was impressively founded by two high school students here in Nova Scotia, Canada). The website description reads as follows: "Deep and enticing, this candle will have you wanting to curl up on a plush couch with a worn, classic book." Notes of candied orange, leather, oakmoss and clove have created a perfect recipe for cozy, inspired writing!

If you enjoy wearing scented products, 'tis the season to update your perfume! I love switching out my summery floral perfume for something richer and more intoxicating when the chilly weather arrives. I'm currently obsessed with *Noir Exquis* by the French brand *L'Artisan Parfumeur*. They describe it as, "An elixir based on the addictive aroma of coffee, blended with comforting scents of orange blossom, maple syrup and candied chestnuts." It smells even more delicious than it sounds.

Visit your closest *Sephora* or department store and have fun sampling different scents. If you are feeling overwhelmed and don't know where to begin, ask for assistance from the sales associate. Warm and sensual notes such as cinnamon, amber and clove, are a good starting point. I'm also a fan of gourmand scents, which include the mouth-watering aromas of coffee, chocolate, vanilla, and caramel.

Follow your nose for an uplifting winter adventure!

17

Blanket Yourself in Warmth

I still love making snow angels, even as an adult. The sight of a fresh, clean blanket of snow is simply irresistible, and I can't help but allow myself to sink into its softness. There is something comforting about being swaddled by nature's quilt of frozen fluff. Lying on my back, face pointing to the sky, I feel safe, supported, and snug.

Soften the blow of winter by blanketing yourself in fluffy comfort. Seek out pleasurable tactile sensations by surrounding yourself with cozy textures this season.

Wrap yourself in the softness of a security blanket by incorporating cozy goodness into your home décor. Soft fuzzy fabrics such as wool, fleece, velvet and faux fur make great companions on a chilly day. Outfit your living spaces with extra throws and blankets so a warm downy embrace is always close at hand. I have a throw draped over every single couch and easy chair in my home this time of year!

If you have hardwood or tile floors, throw down a few extra rugs. I recently placed a sheepskin rug at my bedside. Sinking my feet into its cushiony softness feels delectable when I hop out of bed in the morning.

Consider giving your bed a new winter wardrobe. Pile on an extra quilt or make a switch to fuzzy flannel sheets. (Flannel sheets come in so many cute patterns. You score extra points on the cozy scale for choosing something fun and whimsical.)

Fill your closet with snuggly sweaters and scarves. Natural materials such as wool, cashmere, mohair and alpaca are the best options for keeping you warm. I pretty much live in cashmere turtlenecks from December to the end of February. These luxurious sweaters make me feel elegant and polished, while keeping me toasty with their dreamy softness.

Hot baths are wonderful, until it's time to drain the tub! A cozy robe and slippers will make the transition out of the tub a little easier to bear. One Christmas, my local spa was selling bathrobes by the French skincare brand *Yonka*. I picked one up as a gift for my mother, but shamefully ended up keeping it for myself. It's made of a thick and lush cotton velour and is quite simply divine. It makes the perfect post-bath companion. Treat yourself to the most sumptuous and fluffy robe you can find and envelope yourself in luxury.

Finally, if you share your home with one or more furry friends, invite them up for a snuggle and a little TLC. I own two high-maintenance little poodles, who have the most sumptuously soft hair. I actually look forward to our daily grooming sessions. (Coco loves them, but Junior runs and hides when he sees me coming with the brush.) Working through their mats and running my fingers through their silky fur has a calming effect. Pull out that hairbrush and give your fur baby a beauty treatment. He or she will enjoy the extra attention, and you will benefit from a moment of quiet connection.

Brave the cold by wrapping yourself up in the soft and comforting textures of the season.

18

Chase the Light

everal years ago, my family had the fortune of visiting the city of Arles in the south of France. For those of you not familiar with this area of the world, it was the home of Vincent Van Gogh for a brief period and served as the setting and inspiration for some of his most famous master-pieces—*Starry Night Over the Rhone* and *Café Terrace at Night* included! Visitors of the city can walk the *Van Gogh Circuit*, a self-guided tour that follows his foot-steps and paint strokes to a dozen famous sights.

Van Gogh's time in Provence was a prolific period, resulting in the creation of over three hundred works. This master of impressionism was drawn to the magical light of Provence, as evidenced by these words to his brother Theo, "…the sun has a pale sulphur radiance, and it's soft and charming…". Having visited this area of France, I can confirm, there is indeed something charming and enchanting about the light in this region of the world (not to mention the food, wine, architecture, history, landscape, gardens, shopping…etc.). Is it possible the French government has shrouded the whole region in some fancy, high-tech *Instagram* filter?

On the bleakest of winter days, I find myself daydreaming of the golden Provençal sunlight, yearning for a bit more sparkle in my life. It is human nature, of course, to peer over the fence (or ocean) with envy while turning a blind eye to the blessings right in front of our noses. While lost in longing, I was missing the golden nuggets of beauty my Canadian winter was offering up.

I awakened to this realization one November afternoon while walking around the yard, patiently waiting for my dogs to find that perfect spot to pee. (Apparently, it's not an easy task.) It was late in the day with the sun nestled low in the sky. The trees stood bare, having recently been stripped of their flamboyant and fiery fall foliage. The tamaracks were the only ones still donning amber-colored outfits, hanging on to their needles for just a few more weeks. (The tamarack is one of the few deciduous conifers that loses its needles in the autumn.) Although surrounded by reminders of decay and darkness, I was struck by the golden glow of the late afternoon light. Just as Van Gogh had described, it too was soft, charming, and radiant.

There is a magical quality to the light this time of year when the sun sits lower on the horizon. (It turns out we've got our own *Instagram* filter at play!) Sadly, as the days grow shorter, many people never see the light of day during the winter. When you leave for work before sunrise, and return after sunset, there isn't much opportunity to soak up the sun. Make an effort to peek your head outdoors during daylight hours, even if it is only for a short period of time. Take a walk during lunch or sneak out for a quick coffee run during the afternoon slump. At the very least, position yourself near a window and admire the view from afar.

When venturing outdoors isn't an option, seek out ways to welcome more light and sparkle into your life. Light candles more often and at unexpected times. A candlelit breakfast is the perfect way to add a bit more sparkle to your winter mornings. Christmas lights need not be reserved for the holiday season. String a set of mini lights around one of your potted plants, across the mantle, or along the edge of a bookshelf. My son installed a strip of LED color-changing lights under the frame of his bed. With a dozen different colors to choose from, he can adjust them to suit his every mood!

Adding a mirror to a room is another simple trick to welcome more light into your living spaces. Place a mirror opposite or beside a window. Even on the dimmest of days, it will reflect available daylight to all corners of a room. The bigger the mirror, the more illuminating the effect!

Lastly, sprinkle yourself with a bit of snow fairy dust. Adding some sparkle to your wardrobe is a fun way to capture the light. During the winter, I love wearing clothing with a dash of tasteful and under-stated shimmer. I own a beautiful mohair sweater by one of my favorite French brands, *Sézane*. This cozy navy knit has a fine thread of gold lurex running through the fabric, which produces a subtle glittering effect. Winter is also a great time to wear heavier jewelry. Statement earrings and chunky gold necklaces add vibrancy to any outfit. For a touch of effervescence, spritz your skin or hair with some *Huile Prodigieuse Or* by the French brand *Nuxe*. This dry oil contains tiny shimmering mineral particles that attract the light.

Ignite a love for winter by basking in the golden light around you!

19

Escape

I love chatting with locals whenever I travel. It's the best way to learn about a culture and gain a different perspective. I'm always curious to learn how other countries view Canada on the world stage. On a recent trip to Paris, I struck up a conversation with a young man who mentioned he had spent some time in Canada. Although he enjoyed his stint abroad, he remarked that he much preferred France. What was it about Canada that left a sour taste in his mouth? Our "ten-month winter", as he called it, was just too much to bear.

Clearly, this Frenchman was exaggerating, but sadly he wasn't that far off the mark. It is often joked that we have three winters in Canada—almost winter, winter and still winter. I can still remember my father cooling lobster in a snowbank on Mother's Day each year. (Yes, we celebrate this special day in May like the rest of the world.) It's no wonder many Canadian snowbirds fly south for the winter!

Unfortunately, escaping the snow, sleet and slush for a sunnier destination is not practical or possible for many of us. Thankfully, you don't need a pricy plane ticket or a swanky hotel reservation to escape winter's grasp. Book yourself a virtual vacation to your favorite destination. Armchair travel is a great way to immerse yourself in a new culture and landscape without leaving the comfort of your home. (It's also much kinder on your bank account than the real deal.)

Read a travel-themed book. I particularly enjoy non-fiction, biographical-style books. You can't beat *Under the Tuscan Sun* by Frances Mayes and *A Year in Provence* by Peter Mayle for a European getaway. I've read and reread these classics more times than I can count. I also really enjoyed *Bella Figura* by Kamin Mohammadi, which tells the tale of her year-long stay in Florence.

Cozy up with a TV program or movie set in an exotic location. I probably enjoyed *Emily in Paris* more for the scenery than the ridiculous storyline. *Faraway* is a gem of a little movie that many people have not heard of. Set on a remote and breathtakingly beautiful Croatian island, it is a story of loss, love and new beginnings. The cinematography in this film truly transports you to this foreign land.

Type *armchair travel* into *YouTube's* search bar and take your pick of any destination on the planet. After all these years, and despite his geeky style, I'm still a fan of Rick Steeves. He's been at this game a long time, so definitely knows his stuff! I've watched all his videos on France and found them both entertaining and informative.

What's on your travel itinerary this winter?

20

Feed the Birds

Shopping for men can be a challenge, but not when it comes to my father. There is one standing item on his Christmas wish list that has been there for decades—birdseed! Dad's been feeding the backyard birds for as long as I can remember.

I'll never forget his response when I asked his opinion on whether I should get a dog. Standing in his backyard next to his beloved feeders, he decisively stated, "These birds are the best darn pets I've ever had and the only pet a man needs". Although I chose to ignore his advice, (I ended up with two dogs), he made a good point. While I would never give up my fur babies for a couple of chickadees, backyard birds do have a lot going for them. They are interesting to watch, pleasant to listen to and entertaining to have around. And yes, a bag of sunflower seeds certainly costs much less than my monthly vet bill.

We humans aren't the only ones trying to survive this winter. Adopt some feathered friends this season by hanging a birdfeeder outside your window. Everyone wins in this scenario. The birds will appreciate a trusted and reliable food source, and you will enjoy the company and entertainment they provide. We place our feeder directly outside the living room window so the whole family can admire our daily visitors.

Have fun identifying and learning about the different species of birds that pay your feeder a visit. So far this year we've welcomed chickadees, juncos, blue jays, nuthatches, and a lonely looking woodpecker. I even spotted a barred owl sitting on our porch railing one day. I suspect it wasn't the seeds he had his eye on. (I've been sure to keep Junior on a tight leash ever since.) Keep a bird book close by so you can identify your visitors. My favorite is *The Backyard Birdsong Guide: A Guide to Listening* by Donald Kroodsma. This book comes with a soundtrack, so you can tune into each bird's song with a push of a button.

Would you like to offer your feathered guests a gourmet treat? Hang a couple of suet cakes alongside your seed feeder. These fatty cakes provide an excellent source of high-calorie nutrition, something tiny birdies crave on the coldest of days. Homemade suet cakes are both easy and fun to make. Whipping up a batch is an activity the whole family can take part in. When my kids were little, they loved making this "birdseed playdough" as they called it. If you are interested in giving it a try, I've provided my quick, simple recipe below. Your feathered friends will spread the word that your backyard is the best gig in down. You'll be the squawk of the neighborhood!

Jen's Cozy Up! Bird Cakes

- ✓ 4 cups of water
- ✓ 2 cups of rolled oats
- ✓ 2 cups of lard
- ✓ ½ cup of chunky, natural peanut butter (no added salt or sugar)
- ✓ 1 cup of black oil sunflower seeds
- ✓ ½ cup plain, raw peanuts
- ✓ ¼ cup of thistle seed (also called nyjer seed)
- ✓ 1 ¼ cup of cornmeal
- ✓ ½ cup dried cranberries or raisins

1. Bring the water to a boil and then add the oats. Turn down the heat and simmer until the oats are cooked.
2. Remove the pot from the stove and stir in lard and peanut butter while the oats are still hot.
3. Stir in the remaining ingredients.
4. Let the mixture cool to room temperature.

5. Use your hands to form the "birdseed dough" into small patties or balls. (This is the fun and messy part!)
6. Place the cakes on a baking sheet lined with wax paper, then pop them in the freezer.
7. Once the cakes are frozen, they are ready to be served to your guests!
8. To serve, place your cakes outside on an old plate, or hang them in a mesh onion bag.
9. Store your extra cakes in the freezer.

21

Sit in Quiet

I remember those first few days and weeks of motherhood like they were yesterday. Bringing my firstborn home from the hospital was a magical and awe-inspiring time of my life. Truthfully, it was also a time marked with extreme exhaustion, confusion, and struggle. My mind and body were at odds with one another, playing a game of tug of war. My brain urged me to jump right back into productivity mode. As the dishes and laundry piled up, I felt compelled to act. My bruised and battered body had other plans. Childbirth, breastfeeding, and sleepless nights had taken their toll. All I really wanted to do was curl up in a ball, cuddle my son, and sleep as much as my little bundle of joy would allow!

The age-old advice to, "Sleep when the baby sleeps" is handed out to new mothers for a reason! After my initial resistance, I finally surrendered myself to the season of motherhood I was living at the time. I gave myself grace and let the dishes pile up. I napped often, read novels in bed, and savoured the sweetness of my newborn baby.

You too can surrender to the season. Make a deliberate choice to soften, unwind and loosen your grip this winter. Did you ever consider that our innate urge to slow down during the winter is Mother Nature's gentle way of encouraging us to take a much-needed rest? With the darkness and coldness comes the encouragement to unplug, relax and reflect.

Give yourself the time and space this winter to embrace the quiet and contemplative nature of the season. Engage in introspective activities that feed your soul and spark creativity. The winter is the perfect time to pick up a new craft or tinker in the kitchen. Working with your hands can be incredibly soothing.

Pull out that neglected knitting project and relax into the meditative rhythm of knit one, purl two.

Cozy days at home are tailor-made for inspired writing. *Cozy Up!* is my tenth book in three years. My most productive writing always takes place during the coldest months of the year. While summer beckons me to come out and play, winter invites me to nestle in and indulge in my creative side. Have you always dreamed of writing your own book? There's no time like the present! If you are serious, check out *The Chic Author* by Fiona Ferris. This book kickstarted my own writing journey, and I can't recommend it enough. Even if you aren't interested in making your words public, pull out a journal and write a letter to yourself. There is always so much to learn and discover about ourselves when we put pen to paper.

Are you interested in learning more about the power of mindfulness? The quiet of winter offers a lovely opportunity to welcome a meditation practice into your daily routine. I recently started an eight-week program called *Palouse Mindfulness*. This mindfulness-based stress reduction program can be accessed for

free at www.palousemindfulness.com. It was recom-
mended to me by a trusted mental health professional
as a good starting point for beginners.

Instead of putting up a fight this winter, rest your
weary mind and body. Surrender to the season and
savour the quiet.

22

Get Friendly

I've been subconsciously avoiding this chapter, clearly leaving it to the end. As an introvert, the topic of socializing can be a tough one to unpack. Contrary to popular belief, introverts are not anti-social creatures! For the most part, we are a very friendly, loving group of people who genuinely enjoy connecting with others. One thing that sets us apart from extroverts is our need for greater amounts of alone time. A hefty dose of daily alone time is essential to my well-being and mental health. It allows me to recharge my batteries, work through my problems and tap into my creativity. My husband, the extrovert, is my polar opposite. He thrives in social settings and is invigorated by interactions with others. To simplify it, socializing ignites my husband's energy and extinguishes mine.

The winter season is custom-made for introverts. It provides us with a long list of valid excuses to turn down invitations. It's too cold out. My car won't start. The roads are too icy. I'm already in my pajamas… etc. The long list of available excuses can, however, become a problem. Whether you are introverted, extroverted, or fall somewhere in between, too much time alone isn't good for anyone. Humans are social animals, and the isolating nature of winter can leave many of us feeling lonely.

Even though I crave and savour my alone time, I'm no stranger to loneliness. It seems that so many of life's milestones are marked by periods of loneliness. I struggled with feeling lost and alone when I left home for university, moved to the city for a new job, and left the workforce to stay home with my children. I'm currently teetering on the cusp of a new wave of loneliness, as my fledglings prepare to leave the nest.

No matter where you fall on the social spectrum, resist the urge to hole up like a hermit this winter. Recognize that socializing is an important part of a healthy lifestyle. Tailor your social engagements to suit your personality. If you are an extrovert, you may enjoy group activities. My husband plays hockey two mornings a week and takes part in a fitness boot camp class the other days. (I workout alone in my basement, which suits me perfectly!) Sign yourself up for a winter yoga class, or join a book club. If you love to entertain, why not host a mid-winter potluck at your house with a large group of friends?

When it comes to socializing, introverts tend to stick with smaller groups or one-on-one interactions. I have one particular friend who will often join me on my walks with Coco. Our dogs get along well, and we enjoy the chance to catch up. I also love connecting over tea or coffee with one or two of my closest friends. Visiting a cozy coffee shop gets us out of the house as we enjoy one another's company.

Keep in mind that you don't have to meet face-to-face to connect. While texting and snapping are great for quick hits of contact, I recommend you pick up the phone or *Facetime* for a more meaningful conversation. I text my mother several times I day, but I still rely on our Sunday evening phone calls to truly connect and update each other on our weeks.

Brave the winter in the company of others by staying connected with your tribe!

Bonus

50 Affirmations to Fall in Love with Winter

Well friend, our lovely little rendezvous is soon coming to an end. I hope you have enjoyed our time together as much as I have. I thought I'd leave you with a love letter of sorts. I've created a list of happy winter thoughts to keep the embers of our conversation glowing. Pull out this handy little list any time you come down with a case of the winter blues. Feel free to personalize it as you see fit. (I left a few blank spaces for you at the bottom of the page just for you.)

Repeat after me, "I love winter because…"

1. My home is my winter retreat. I feel warm, safe and at peace as soon as I walk through the door.
2. The cold temperature brings a rosy glow to my cheeks, making me look and feel vibrant.
3. My skin is enjoying a break from the bright summer sun. It is feeling plump and hydrated after switching to a decadent new moisturizer.
4. The crisp air in the morning fills me with energy and makes me feel alive.
5. Switching my breakfast to a warm bowl of oatmeal brings a sense of comfort to cool mornings.
6. My morning cup of coffee is pure bliss. It warms me up from the inside out.
7. I just treated myself to a new pair of figure skates! After twenty years off the ice, I'm so excited to lace them up and revisit my childhood passion.
8. Starting my day with a morning meditation leaves me feeling grounded.

9. My dark red lipstick shows off my smile and makes my teeth look pearly white.

10. It felt so good to chop off my sun-damaged hair. I'm entering the new season with a new haircut and a fresh outlook.

11. I love walking in the woods this time of year without being pestered by mosquitoes and black flies.

12. I enjoy stacking firewood. It's meditative and great exercise.

13. The darker evenings make the house feel cozy and snug.

14. I love the sound of fallen leaves crunching beneath my feet.

15. Exercising in the cooler temperatures is so refreshing.

16. My houseplants make my home feel alive and cozy on the darkest of days.

17. Warm stews and soups on the menu make me feel nourished and satisfied.

18. The glow from the woodstove is warm and comforting.

19. It feels luxurious to wrap myself up in my fuzzy mohair cardigans.

20. Spicy-scented candles make the house smell delicious.

21. I'm inspired to learn and take on new projects this time of year.

22. It's fun to play around with scarves this time of year. I love the cozy feeling of having something soft and luxurious around my neck.

23. After the hot sticky summer, it feels great to slip on my favorite jeans again. They still fit like a glove.

24. As the weather cools off, I love switching out my wardrobe and pulling out all my favorite items from last year. It feels like Christmas to see them again.

25. I love dressing in the dark, rich jewel tones of the season. These luxurious hues make me feel chic and sophisticated.

26. I'm not worried about hurricane season and winter storms. I know our house is solid and we are well prepared for power and water outages.

27. Cleaning up the garden beds and yard in the fall is rewarding. I feel like I'm tucking my plants in for the winter and sending them to dreamland.

28. I feel motivated to tackle the projects that were put on the back burner during the summer.

29. As I observe death and dormancy taking place around me, I feel grateful to be alive.

30. I enjoy wearing more dramatic eye makeup and not worrying about my mascara smudging in the humidity.

31. The golden light of the late afternoon is enchanting.

32. I'm so happy I finally finished up those old crafting projects. Working with my hands feeds my soul.

33. I savour the cozy warmth of my bed on dark and chilly mornings.

34. I love cozy Sunday mornings with PJs and pancakes.

35. I love watching the chickadees flit outside my window at the feeder. It feels good

knowing I'm helping them survive this frigid winter.

36. Afternoon naps on lazy Sundays feel decadent and delicious.

37. Shovelling snow is great exercise. I feel my body getting stronger with each storm!

38. My winter reading list keeps me company on dark cold nights.

39. I adore watching movies wrapped in my faux fur blanket. It feels delectable against my skin.

40. I look forward to tucking myself in for the night with a good book and a cup of calming tea.

41. An early sunset allows me to dine in the glow of candlelight.

42. Winter calls for extra snuggling on the couch with my loved ones.

43. My morning workout keeps me warm all day long.

44. I love the heady scent of my winter perfume. It makes me feel sensual and mysterious.

45. My winter coat looks fabulous on me. I get compliments everywhere I go!

46. Even though it's cold, I enjoy getting out of the house and meeting a friend for a coffee. It's nice to connect with someone I care about.

47. I'm prepared for any weather winter throws at me. I've learned to layer up and never miss a day outside.

48. The solitude of winter calms my mind.

49. The blanket of fresh fallen snow sparkles in the sunlight and dazzles me with its beauty.

50. I've grown to love and look forward to winter. It is truly a magical time of the year.

51.

52.

53.

54.

55.

A Note from the Author

*T*hank you so much for joining me for this cozy little chat. It's been lovely connecting with you and sharing my vision of a winter wonderland. I hope I've convinced you that despite its harshness, winter offers its own unique brand of magic.

Be dazzled by the beauty of winter! Enter the season with intention and a sense of gratitude for the gifts it has to offer. Wrap yourself up in the cozy goodness of fuzzy sweaters, tasty soups, good books, and long chats. Savour the deliciousness of serene landscapes, cozy nights, golden light and heart-warming moments of reflection and connection. Glide through the season with a sense of hope, enthusiasm, comfort and contentment.

If you enjoyed this book and my writing style, I have many other titles that would make great additions to your cozy winter reading list! My books can all be found on *Amazon* in both paperback and eBook format. I love exploring the concept of elevating the experience of everyday life. As such, my writing covers a wide range of lifestyle topics including personal style, home décor, household management, travel, fitness, health, nutrition, personal finances, attitude… and so much more!

I also have a little favor to ask of you! If you enjoyed *Cozy Up!* please take a quick moment to leave a review on *Amazon.* As a self-published author, reviews are incredibly helpful and greatly appreciated. Not only do they provide me with valuable feedback, but they help me connect with my readers and spread the word about my writing.

Thank you again for our lovely time together. I'm sending sunny thoughts your way and wish you a fabulous, cozy winter season filled with warmth, love, light and sparkle!

Much love,

Jennifer

Other Books by Jennifer Melville

Elevate the Everyday:
Actions and Ideas to Enhance the Experience of Daily Life

Elevate Your Personal Style:
Inspiration for the Everyday Woman

Elevate Your Health:
*Inspiration and Motivation to Embrace and
Maintain a Healthy Lifestyle*

Elevate Your Life at Home:
Inspiring Ideas to Add Joy, Peace and Magic to Your Homelife

Elevate Your Money Mindset:
Approach Your Finances With Positivity, Confidence and Enthusiasm

Preloved Chic:
Stylish Secrets to Elevate Your Wardrobe With Second-Hand Fashion

Paris in my Panties:
Live Your Best (French Inspired) Life

Seashells in my Pocket:
50 Ways to Live a Beach Inspired Life

Blissful Christmas:
Glide Through the Holidays With Less Effort and More Joy

About the Author

Jennifer Melville is a self-published author. She decided to embark on a writing career because she wanted to tap into a community of like-minded individuals who share in her enthusiasm for living well and seeking ways to elevate daily life. She is a professional accountant by trade, who approaches life with an analytical and observant mind. Jennifer has been exploring the concept of elevating the everyday for over twenty years. She is passionate about family, health, fitness, fashion, nutrition, nature and all the beauty life has to offer.

Jennifer lives by the sea in beautiful Nova Scotia, Canada with her husband, two sons and little poodles Coco and Junior.

You can connect with her by email, on her blog, or on her Instagram page.

jenniferlynnmelville@gmail.com

www.theelevatedeveryday.com

www.instagram.com/the.elevated.everyday

Printed in Great Britain
by Amazon

32355470R00067